María Antonia Meroño Saura
Pilar Pacheco López
María Rodríguez Romero

NUTRITION AND AMYOTROPHIC LATERAL SCLEROSIS

María Antonia Meroño Saura
Pilar Pacheco López
María Rodríguez Romero

NUTRITION AND AMYOTROPHIC LATERAL SCLEROSIS

Effect of different foods and nutrients on the risk and progression of amyotrophic lateral sclerosis

ScienciaScripts

Imprint

Any brand names and product names mentioned in this book are subject to trademark, brand or patent protection and are trademarks or registered trademarks of their respective holders. The use of brand names, product names, common names, trade names, product descriptions etc. even without a particular marking in this work is in no way to be construed to mean that such names may be regarded as unrestricted in respect of trademark and brand protection legislation and could thus be used by anyone.

Cover image: www.ingimage.com

This book is a translation from the original published under ISBN 978-3-659-09485-9.

Publisher:
Sciencia Scripts
is a trademark of
Dodo Books Indian Ocean Ltd. and OmniScriptum S.R.L publishing group

120 High Road, East Finchley, London, N2 9ED, United Kingdom
Str. Armeneasca 28/1, office 1, Chisinau MD-2012, Republic of Moldova, Europe
Printed at: see last page
ISBN: 978-620-6-11750-6

INDEX

SUMMARY

Amyotrophic lateral sclerosis (ALS) is a neurodegenerative disease of unknown cause, which presents with weakness in the limbs or difficulties in speaking or swallowing, which may be associated with a high nutritional risk. There is currently no cure, so it is approached in a multidisciplinary manner with both pharmacological and non-pharmacological interventions, including nutritional interventions. The aim of the present study was to elucidate the relationship between diet composition and the risk of developing ALS and the evolution of ALS once established. A review of the scientific literature on the effects of different dietary components on ALS was carried out. The descriptors used were: "diet", "nutrition", "food habit", "eating habit", "lifestyle", "food", "amyotrophic lateral sclerosis" and "als". Twenty articles assessing the effects of different nutrients and dietary characteristics on the risk of developing ALS and its progression were included. After data extraction, we observed nutrients and foods that promoted the development of ALS (red meat), decreased the risk (antioxidants) and had no effect (mercury), foods and nutrients that promoted the progression of the disease (intake deficit) and reduced it (antioxidants). In conclusion, dietary composition and intake of certain micronutrients and foods appear to influence the initial development and progression of ALS, however, controlled studies with larger samples comparing different dietary patterns are needed to locate their true role in the disease.

Keywords: amyotrophic lateral sclerosis, nutrition, nutrient, food, risk, prognosis

INTRODUCTION

Amyotrophic lateral sclerosis (ALS) is a neurodegenerative disease that mainly affects the motor system, although it is also accompanied by extra-motor manifestations (1). Clinically, it shows a combination of symptoms and signs related to the destruction of upper and lower motor neurons, as well as neuronal degeneration in other regions such as the brainstem and spinal cord. (1). Typical upper symptoms and signs are weakness, hyperreflexia and spasticity. The lower ones are amyotrophy and fasciculations.

The incidence of ALS worldwide is estimated at 0.6-3.8/100000 persons/year, while in Europe it is estimated at 2.1-3.8/100000 persons/year, and is expected to increase in the coming years. (2).

The causes of the disease are still unknown. Scientific literature considers different factors such as the influence of viruses, toxins, glutamate- and homocysteine-mediated excitotoxicity, mitochondrial dysfunction, oxidative stress, alterations of the cytoskeleton and defects in axonal transport, altered RNA and DNA metabolism or immunodeficiency. (3). The role of possible chronic inflammation has also been suggested. (3). Other risk factors could be older age, male sex, body mass index, smoking and dyslipidaemias, mainly at the expense of LDL (3). Not to mention an autosomal dominant genetic inheritance due to well-known genetic mutations (3).

In terms of diagnosis, the standard criteria for ALS were established in 1991, and are the *El Escorial Criteria*, revised in 1997 and renamed the modified *El Escorial Criteria*. (4). Although the essential requirements for the diagnosis of ALS are defined by these criteria, they have a low clinical accuracy (4). In 2008, electrodiagnostic studies, known as the *Awaji Criteria*, were included in the clinical procedure to allow earlier and more accurate assessment of the diagnosis of ALS (4). These criteria take into account the presence or absence of various neuronal alterations and classify patients into 4 levels of diagnostic certainty, namely clinically definite, probable, probable laboratory supported and possible ALS (5). (5). However, the application of these defined feature sets is still insufficient to rule out other similar and related diseases. (4).

Once the disease has been diagnosed, different scales are used to measure the severity and progression of symptoms and signs, most notably the *Amyotrophic Lateral Sclerosis Functional Rating Scale (ALSFRS)*. This easy-to-use scale assesses the patient's disability by areas: gross motor tasks, fine motor tasks, bulbar functions and respiratory function. (6).

As mentioned above, ALS usually manifests with weakness in the limbs or difficulty in speaking or swallowing. Partly because of these symptoms, the Ethics Working Group of the Spanish Society of Nutrition (SENPE) concluded that the clinical features of ALS carry a high nutritional risk (7). During the course of the disease a large percentage of patients develop malnutrition of any degree, occurring in 16-55% of patients at the time of diagnosis (7). The effects of ALS on nutritional status are due to anorexia related to the patient's psychosocial situation and possible drug-related adverse effects; constipation related to abdominal and pelvic muscle weakness, associated with decreased intake; impaired chewing and swallowing in bulbar ALS; increased catabolism in the early stages of the disease; and refusal to eat which may be associated with the onset of dementia (7). (7). The SENPE work also elucidated that there are several markers of nutritional status that can be used as a prognostic factor for the disease, such as low body mass index and increased weight loss, which are associated with worse disease outcome. Body composition is also related to disease progression, a decrease in both free muscle mass and fat mass are associated with a worse prognosis. (7,8).

In terms of treatment, there is currently no curative therapy, so the cornerstone of disease management remains a multidisciplinary approach, which has a positive effect on both patient satisfaction and outcomes. On the one hand, we have symptomatic treatment of the different manifestations, including pharmacological and non-pharmacological interventions. In terms of pharmacological treatment, the only drugs that have managed to prolong patient survival by a few months have been *riluzole*, whose mechanism of action is the blockade of glutamate release, and *edaravone*, which prevents oxidative damage from free radicals (9,10).

In terms of non-pharmacological measures, neurorehabilitation treatment and nutritional measures stand out. Focusing on the latter, in the review by López-Gómez JJ et al, it was observed that patients diagnosed with ALS who followed a specific nutritional protocol had a better evolution of body composition and a higher survival rate. (8). Among the nutritional measures, they highlighted: a caloric and protein intake adapted to the patient's evolution, modification of the texture of food and liquids, postural manoeuvres to facilitate swallowing and the use of adapted crockery, the use of hyperproteic, hypercaloric supplements with different proportions of carbohydrates and fat, omega-3 (W-3), enteral or parenteral nutrition, depending on the stage of the disease (8).

Due to the increasing incidence of the disease, the absence of effective treatments and the influence of nutritional status on the prognosis and evolution of the disease, it is necessary to establish dietary guidelines to optimise nutritional treatment, seeking the greatest benefit for the patient. Therefore, the aim of the present study was to evaluate the relationship between diet composition and the risk of developing the disease as well as its influence on the prognosis and evolution of amyotrophic lateral sclerosis.

In order to evaluate the relationship between diet composition and ALS risk and its evolution, a systematic review of the literature was carried out with defined search parameters in different databases as defined in the material and methods section. In the results section, the most relevant data from the included studies have been presented, whose results and limitations have been analysed and compared with other published studies in the discussion section. Finally, after examining the available data, the effect of nutrients and diet on ALS has been recapitulated and concluded.

OBJECTIVE

- The main objective of the present study was to evaluate the relationship between diet composition and the risk of developing ALS, as well as its influence on the prognosis and evolution of ALS.

- The secondary objectives were: to assess the effects of calorie intake, food groups, and macronutrients and micronutrients on the prognosis and outcome of ALS.

MATERIAL AND METHODS

A systematic literature review of the scientific literature on the effects of diet composition on the progression of ALS has been carried out.

Search strategy

Initially, the selection of key words for the search of health sciences descriptors (DeCS) was carried out using the Virtual Health Library (VHL) website. The descriptors used, both in English and Spanish, were: *diet, nutrition, food habit, eating habit, lifestyle, food, amyotrophic lateral sclerosis or als*. Using these and the Boolean operators "AND" and "OR", a search for articles was carried out, as described in table 1, in the databases Medline complete, VHL Regional Portal, Lilacs, Scielo and Cuiden, taking into account the inclusion and exclusion criteria described in table 2.

Database	Search string	Results found
Medline Complete	diet" or "nutrition" or "food habit" or "eating habit" or "lifestyle" or "food" AND "amyotrophic lateral sclerosis" or "als" AND "amyotrophic lateral sclerosis" or "als".	1096
VHL Regional Portal	diet" or "nutrition" or "food habit" or "eating habit" or "lifestyle" or "food" AND "amyotrophic lateral sclerosis" or "als" AND "amyotrophic lateral sclerosis" or "als".	726
Scielo	diet" or "nutrition" or "food habit" or "eating habit" or "lifestyle" or "food" AND "amyotrophic lateral sclerosis" or "als" AND "amyotrophic lateral sclerosis" or "als".	19
Lilacs	"diet" or "nutrition" or "food habit" or "eating habit" or "lifestyle" or "food" AND "amyotrophic lateral sclerosis" or "als".	17

Table 1. Bibliographic search process

Inclusion criteria	Exclusion criteria

· Articles published in the last five years, i.e. between 2013 and 2022.	· Articles published before 2013.
· Language: Spanish and English.	· Language other than English or Spanish.
· Full text available.	· Full text not available.
· Articles related to the objectives of this work.	· Articles whose topics are not related to the objectives of this work.
	· Clinical cases, theses, letters to the editor or systematic reviews or animal studies.

Table 2. Inclusion and exclusion criteria

The search yielded a total of 1858 studies. Duplicate studies were checked before reading the title and abstract. After this review, 1209 studies were excluded because they were systematic reviews, clinical cases, animal studies or did not meet the study objectives. Of the remaining 37, 18 were excluded after reading the full paper, 1 because the results of the paper had not been published, 4 because the study variable was the presence of Beta-methylamino-L-alanine in oysters consumed by ALS patients, and 13 because the intervention consisted of supplements of different categories, and not dietary intake. The remaining articles were examined and the quality of the rest was analysed by critical reading with the help of CASPe, discarding one article because it only analysed hydration status, and another because it included patients with other neurological disorders in addition to ALS.

Finally, the sample for this work consisted of 20 articles. Figure 1 shows the selection process. The processing and study of the bibliographic reference data was carried out using Microsoft Office Word® and the Zotero® database.

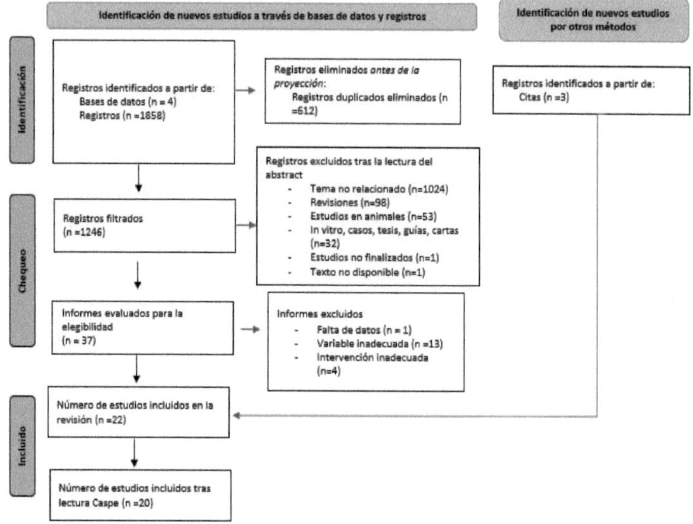

Illustration 1Flowchart for item selection

RESULTS

Following the literature review, a total of 20 articles related to the objectives set out in this study were obtained. Table 3 shows the main characteristics of the articles included.

TITLE AND AUTHORS	YEAR	MAGAZINE	PATIENTS	TYPE OF STUDY	FOLLOW-UP	FACTOR OF INTEREST	EVIDENCE
Fat-rich versus carbohydrate-rich nutrition in ALS: a randomised controlled study **Dorst J, Doenz J, Kandler K, Dreyhaupt J, Tumani H, Witzel S, et al** (11).	2022	Journal of Neurology, Neurosurgery & Psychiatry	Patients diagnosed with Definite, probable or possible ALS N= 64	Clinical trial prospective randomised trial of groups parallels	4 weeks	Group 1: Supplement high-calorie fatty (HCFS). Group 2: Supplement fatty acids (UHCFS). Group 3: Supplement of ultra-caloric carbohydrates (UHCCS) Group 4: No supplement	1b

Amyotrophic Lateral Sclerosis Risk, Family Income, and Fish Consumption Estimates of Mercury and Omega-3 PUFAs in the United States **Hoffman HI, Bradley WG, Chen CY, Pioro EP, Stommel EW, Andrew AS** (12)	2021	Internation Journal of Environment al Research and Public Health	Patients over 21 years of age diagnosed with probable or definite ALS N= 165 cases N= 330 controls	Case-control study	4 years Diagnosis (2016-2020)	Annual consumption of annual mercury and acid intakes polyunsaturated fatty acids omega-3 (PUFA)	3b

Comparison Mercury of exposure from Seafood consumption and Dental Amalgam Fillings in People with and without Amyotrophic Lateral Sclerosis (ALS): An International Online Case-Control Study. **Parkin Kullmann J, Pamphlett R. A** (13)	2018	International Journal of Environment al Research and Public Health	Patients who self-report being diagnosed with ALS N= 401 cases N= 452 controls	Case study - international monitoring	2 years Surveys (2015-2017)	Exposure to mercury through consumption seafood	3b
Relationship between Dietary Fiber Intake and the Prognosis of Amytrophic Lateral Sclerosis in Korea. **Yu H, Kim SH, Noh MY, Lee S, Park Y** (14)	2020	Nutrients	Patients diagnosed with probable or possible ALS N=272	Descriptive observational study	9 years (March 2011- September 2020)	Intake of different types of dietary fibre by tertiles	2b

| Effect of high-caloric nutrition on serum neurofilament light chain levels in amyotrophic lateral sclerosis. **Dorst J, Dreyhaupt J, Witzel S, Weishaupt JH, Kassubek J, et al.** (15) | 2020 | Journal of Neurology, Neurosurgery & Psychiatry | Patients with definite, probable or probable ALS N=29 intervention N= 41 placebo | Multicentre, randomised, double-blind, parallel-group, multicentre clinical trial. | 18 months + 14 days | Hypercaloric fat diet (405kcal extra fat per day) vs. placebo | 1b |
| Effect of High-Caloric Nutrition on Survival in Amyotrophic Lateral Sclerosis. **Ludolph AC, Dorst J, Dreyhaupt J, Weishaupt JH, Kassubek J** (16) | 2020 | Annals of Neurology | Patients with definite, probable or possible ALS N= 104 intervention N= 103 placebo | 1:1 randomised, double-blind, multicentre, double-blind, parallel-group clinical trial | 18 months + 14 days | Hypercaloric fat diet (405kcal extra fat per day) vs. placebo. | 1b |

Association between macronutrient intake and amyotrophic lateral sclerosis prognosis. **Kim B, Jin Y, Kim SH, Park Y** (17)	2020	Nutritional Neuroscience	Patients diagnosed with ALS N= 148	Descriptive observational study	6 years (2011- 2017)	Macronutrient intake	2b
Coffee, tea, and caffeine intake and amyotrophic lateral sclerosis mortality in a pooled analysis of eight prospective cohort studies. **Petimar J, O'Reilly É, Adami H - O., Brandt PA, Buring J, English DR, et al** (18)	2019	European Journal of Neurology	Patients diagnosed with ALS N=545	Pooled analysis of prospective studies of cohorts	12-24 years	Caffeine consumption	2a

Title / Authors	Year	Journal	Population	Study design	Duration	Variables	
Coffee and Tea Consumption Impact on Amyotrophic Lateral Sclerosis Progression: A Multicenter Cross-Sectional Study. **Cucovici A, Ivashynka A, Fontana A, Russo S, Mazzini L, Mandrioli J, et al. (19)**	2021	Frontiers in Neurology	Patients diagnosed with ALS N= 145	Cross-sectional descriptivomulticentric study	4 years (October 2016- January 2020)	Consumption of tea or coffee	4
Amyotrophic lateral sclerosis and food intake. **Pupillo E, Bianchi E, Chiò A, Casale F, Zecca C, Tortelli R, et al (20)**	2018	Amyotrophic Lateral Sclerosis and Frontotemporal Degeneration	Patients newly diagnosed with ALS N= 212 cases N= 212 controls	Study case-control study	4 years (2011- 2015)	Daily intake of macronutrients, micronutrients, fatty acids and total energy	3b

| Dietary intake and zinc status in amyotrophic lateral sclerosis. **Lopes da Silva HF, Araújo Brito AN, Silva de Freitas EP, Teixeira Dourado Jr. ME, Sena-Evangelista KCM, Leite Lais L** (21) | 2017 | Hospital Nutrition | Patients diagnosed with of ALS N= 20 cases N= 37 controls | Study single -centre case- control study | 1 year (2015-2016) | Dietary intakes of macronutrients, energy, fibre and zinc consumption | 3b |

The Impact of Lifetime Alcohol and Cigarette Smoking Loads on Amyotrophic Lateral Sclerosis Progression: A Cross-Sectional Study. **Cucovici A, Fontana A, Ivashynka A, Russo S, Renna V, Mazzini L, et al** (22)	2021	Life	Patients wit h a clinical diagnosis of ALS N= 241	Descriptivom ulticentric cross- sectional study	4years (October 2016- January 2020)	Tobacco and alcohol exposure	4

Association Between Dietary Intake and Function in amyotrophic Lateral Sclerosis. **Nieves JW, Gennings C, Factor-Litvak P, Hupf J, Singleton J, Sharf V, et al** (23)	2016	JAMA neurology	Patients with a diagnosis of ALS and the onset of the disease symptoms for less than 18 months N= 302 patients	Cross-sectional descriptivom ulticentric study	5 years (March 2008-February 2017)	Intake of food groups and micronutrients — 4
Association between nutritional status and disease severity using the amyotrophic lateral sclerosis (ALS) functional rating scale in ALS patients. **Park Y, Park J, Kim Y, Baek H, Kim SH** (24)	2015	Nutrition	Patients diagnosed with ALS N= 193	Descriptive cross-sectional study	1 year (October 2012-December 2013)	Intake of different food groups 4

Dietary ω-3 Polyunsaturated Fatty Acid Intake and Risk for Amyotrophic Lateral Sclerosis. **Fitzgerald KC, O'Reilly ÉJ, Falcone GJ, Mc Cullough ML, Park Y, Kolonel LN et al. (25)**	2014	JAMA Neurology	Patients diagnosed with ALS confirmed by the neurologist N= 995	Pooled analysis of 5 prospective cohort studies	9-24 years	Consumption of omega-6 and omega-3 polyunsaturated fatty acids	2a

Effect of Presymptomatic Body Mass Index and Consumption of Fat and Alcohol on Amyotrophic Lateral Sclerosis. **Huisman MHB, Seelen M, Doormaal PTC van, Jong SW de, Vries JHM de, Kooi AJ van der, et al** (26)	2015	JAMA Neurology	Patients with new diagnosis of possible, probable or definite ALS N= 674 cases N= 2093 controls	Study case-control	4years (January-2006- April 2013)	Fat and alcohol intake	3b
Intakes of caffeine, coffee and tea and risk of amyotrophic lateral sclerosis: Results from five cohort studies. **Fondell E, O'Reilly ÉiJ, Fitzgerald KC, Falcone GJ, Kolonel LN, Park Y, et al.** (27)	2015	Amyotrophic Lateral Sclerosis and Frontotemporal Degeneration	Patients with a diagnosis of ALS N= 1279	Pooled analysis of 5 prospective cohort studies	18 years	Caffeine, coffee and tea intake	2a

Dietary intake of fruits and beta-carotene is negatively associated with amyotrophic lateral sclerosis risk in Koreans: A case- control study. **Jin Y, Oh K, Oh S il, Baek H, Kim SH, Park Y.** (28)	2014	Nutritional neuroscience	Patients diagnosed with ELA N= 72 cases N= 72 controls	Case- control study	1 year (March 2011- February 2012)	Fruit and beta-carotene intake	3b
Magnesium intake and risk of amyotrophic lateral sclerosis: Results from five large cohort studies. **Fondell E, O'Reilly ÉJ, Fitzgerald KC, Falcone GJ, McCullough ML, Park Y, et al** (29)	2013	Amyotrophic Lateral Sclerosis and Frontotempor al Degeneration	Patients with a diagnosis of ALS N= 1093	Pooled analysis of 5 prospective cohort studies	15 years	Magnesium intake	2a

Intakes of vitamin C and carotenoids and risk of amyotrophic lateral sclerosis: Pooled results from 5 cohort studies: carotenoids and ALS. **Fitzgerald KC, O'Reilly ÉJ, Fondell E, Falcone GJ, McCullough ML, Park Y, et al (30)**	2013	Annals of Neurology	Patients with a diagnosis of ALS N= 1153	Combined analysis of 5 prospective cohort studies	Median of 11 years	Intake of carotenoids and vitamin C	2a

Table 3. Selected titles

With regard to the methodological characteristics of the studies, different types of studies were found, with very similar inclusion and exclusion criteria in all the studies, although with certain nuances.

Three randomised clinical trials (RCTs), five pooled analyses of cohort studies, six case-control studies, four descriptive cross-sectional studies and two descriptive observational studies were included.

The type of patient included is shown in table 4. It was noted that there were differences in the papers between the stage of disease included (possible, probable or definitive), and how the diagnosis was made.

Pupillo et al, Lopes Da Silva et al, Hoffman et al, Jin et al and Nieves et al, used the Escorial or Awaji Criteria to confirm the diagnosis. In the work of Huisman et al, Fitzgerald et al. and Fondell et al, the presence or absence of ALS was reported by patients in various questionnaires, and the diagnosis was then confirmed by medical history request or confirmation by the neurologist. In addition, they included patients from the total pool with clinical coding ICD-9 335.2 or ICD-10 G12.2 (motor neuron disease). Parkin et al. followed the same methodology, but without subsequent confirmation of the diagnosis.

Exclusion criteria were common in some studies, in the three randomised clinical trials, in the works of Pupillo et al, Kim et al, Yu et al, Cucovici et al and Park et al, patients with SGA, tracheostomy or non-invasive ventilation for more than 23h per day or with other neurodegenerative pathologies were excluded, as well as those who did not sign the informed consent. In the work of Dorst et al. and Kim et al., patients taking any type of supplement were also excluded. In the work of Petimar et al, patients who died within the first two years were also excluded because of possible interference with the results. Unlike the others, Parkin et al. excluded patients older than 40 years.

Regarding sample size, in one of the RCTs the sample size was statistically pre-specified to obtain a statistical power of 80%, in the remaining two RCTs the sample size depended on the availability of patients, without being estimated by any calculation.

In the pooled analyses of cohort studies, the studies by Fondell et al, and Fitzgerald et al, were based on the population of the following five cohort studies: the Nurses' Health Study, the Health Professionals Follow-up Study, the Cancer Prevention Study II Nutrition Cohort, the Multiethnic Cohort Study, and the National Institutes of Health-AARP Diet and Health Study, with a total population of 1010000 patients. The remaining work was based on 8 prospective studies covering a total population of 351565 patients, from which patients meeting the inclusion criteria were selected.

In the case-control studies, only in one paper were cases matched with controls (N=72). In the other studies, the number of controls was much higher than the number of cases. For their selection , Hoffman et al. selected you by mail with a 2:1 ratio by propensity score matching. Jin et al. matched patients 1:1 with controls, with no significant differences between the two groups. In the other papers, the method of control selection was not specified.

The duration of symptom duration (months, years...) differed between the inclusion criteria of the different publications.

Characteristics of the participants

All studies involved adult patients diagnosed with ALS. Table 4 shows the main characteristics of the patients included in each study:

Author	Sex	Age	P
Dorst et al (11)	Group 1 (n=15): 2 (13.3%) females and 13 (86.7%) males Group2 (n=16): 3 (18.7%) females and 13 (81.3%) males Group 3 (n= 17): 7 (41.2%) women and 10 (58.8%) men. Group4 (n=16): 6 (37.5%) women and 10 (62.5%) men Total: 18 women and 46 men	Group 1 (n=15): 61.5±7.5 Group 2 (n=16): 57.6±7.0 Group 3 (n= 17): 59.9±9.5 Group 4 (n=16): 62.1±10.5 Total: 60.3±8.7	P age: 0.49 P sex: 0.23 Remaining characteristics (weight, BMI, disease variables...) P>0.05

Hoffma n HI et al (12)	Controls: 132 (40%) females and 198 (60%) males Cases: 71 (43%) women and 95 (57%) men.	Controls: <50 years: 23 (7%), 50-65 years: 159 (48.2%), 65- 75 years old: 115 (34.8%), >75 years old years: 33 (10%) Cases: <50 years: 13 (7.9%), 50-65 years old: 76 (46,1%), 65- 75 years old: 58 (35.2%), >75 years old years: 18 (10.9%)	P age: 0.96 P sex: 0.58 Family history of ALS p<0.001 All other characteristics (race, disease characteristics) characteristics) P>0.05
Parki n JA et al (13)	Controls: 322 (71.24%) females and 130 (28.76%) males Cases: 149women (37.16%) and 252 (62.84%) men.	Controls: 57.3 ± 10.4 (40-89 years) Cases: 61.5 ± 9.2 (40-87 years).	P age <0.001 P age men >0.05 P age women <0.001
Yu et al (14)	T1: 39 (43.33%) women and 51 (56.7%) men T2: 41 (45.05%) women and 50 (54.9%) men T3: 47 (51.65%) women and 44 (48.4%) men Total: 127 (46.7%) women and 145 (53.3%) men	T1: 55.29 ± 10.62 at symptom onset T2: 54.76 ± 1.66 at onset of symptoms T3: 52.99 ± 10.20 at onset of symptoms Total: 54.34 ± 10.50 at symptom onset.	P age: 0.404 P sex: 0.496 P smoking, drinking IIMC >0.05 P exercise: 0.001 P disease progression <0.001

Dorst et al (15)	Intervention group: Women 51% and men 49%. Placebo group: Women 35% and men 65%. Total: Women 43% and men 57%.	Intervention group: 62.6 ± 11.4 years Placebo group: 62.8 ± 10.1 years Total: 62.7 ± 10.7 years	P age: 0.92 P sex: 0.11 Other characteristics (BMI, disease characteristics) P >0.05
Ludolph AC et al (16)	Intervention group: 41 (40.2%) and 61 (59.8%) men Placebo group : 39 (39.4%) females and 60 (60.6%) males Total: 80 (39.8%) females and 121 (60.2%) males	Intervention group: 62.4±11.0 Control group: 62.4 ± 10.6 Total: 62.4 ± 10.8	Not specified
Kim B et al(17)	54 (36.5%) women and 94 (63.1% men)	55.52±9.70 at symptom onset	Not specified
Petimar Jet at (18)	328 (60.18%) Women and 217 (39.82%) Men	Women: 154 between 55-69 years 36 between 27-76 years 27 between 55-74 years 51 between 40-76 years Men 42 between 45-89 years 18 between 30-49 years old 74 between 45-79 years old 28 between 27-75 years 83 between 55-69 years 32 between 55-74 years	P sex >0.25 P non-linearity >0.1

Cucovic i A et al (19)	Non-users: 16 (47.1%) women and 18 (52.9%) men.	Non-consumers: 64.3 ± 11.3	P age former consumers: 0.227
	Former users 1-3 cups: 5 (41.7%) females and 7 (58.3%) males	Former consumers 1-3 cups: 64.6 ± 12.4	P age of current consumers: 0.415
	Former consumers 4-8 cups: 4 (40%) women and 6 (60%) men.	Former consumers 4-8 cups: 58.9 ± 10.1	P age former consumers vs non-consumers: 0.403
	Current Consumers 1-3 cups: 52 (37.7%) females and 86 (62.3%) males	Current Consumers 1-3 cups: 62.5 ± 11.3	P age new consumers vs non-consumers: 0.232
	Current consumers 4-8 cups: 15 (36.6%) women and 26 (63.4%) men.	Current consumers 4-8 cups: 60.9 ± 9.3	Psexo former consumers: 1
			Psex current consumers: 1
			P sex former consumers vs non-consumers: 0.785
			P sex new consumers vs. non-consumers: 0.339
			P BMI, Country, age of symptom onset, education >0.05

Pupillo et al (20)	Cases: 94 (44.3%) females and 118 (55.7%) males. Controls: Equal	Cases: <50 years: 25 Between 50-54 years old: 22 55-59 years old: 24 60-64 years old: 42 65-69 years old: 44 Between 70-74 years: 30 >75 years: 25 Controls: <50 years: 24 Between 50-54 years: 20 55-59 years old: 19 60-64 years old: 37 65-69 years old: 48 Between 70-74 years old: 33 >75 years: 31	P other characteristics >0.05
Lopes HE et al (21)	Controls: 24 (65%) women and 13 (35%) men Cases: 11 (55%) females and 9 (45%) males.	Controls: 42.48 ± 11.21 Cases: 54.86 ± 13.95	P age: 0.008 (SIGNIFICANT) P sex: 0.571 P BMI >0.05
Cucovic i A et al (22)	Slow progression : 28 (34.6%) females and 53 (65.4%) males Average progression : 36 (45%) women and 44 (55%) men Rapid progression : 32 (40%) women and 48 (60%) men Total: 96 (39.8%) women and 145 (60.2%) men	Slow progression: 59.8 ± 12.3 Average progression: 63.6 ± 10.4 Rapid progression: 63.9 ± 9.8 Total: 62.4 ± 11.0	P age: 0.032 P sex: 0.401 P education, BMI >0.05 *Considered significant difference P<0.01* *signif icant difference P<0.01*

Nevis JW et al (23)	124 (41.06%) Women and 178 (59.8%) Men	63.2 years (55.5-68)	No significant differences in sex, age or race
Park Y et al (24)	Low ALSFRS-R score: 42 (64.4%) men Mean ALSFRS-R score: 36 (59%) men High ALSFRS-R score: 42 (62.7%) men	Low ALSFRS-R score: 53.91 ± 1.34 years Score Mean ALSFRS-R: 57.44 ± 1.26 years High ALSFRS-R score: 53.75 ± 1.29 years	P age: 0.085 P sex: 0.806 P characteristics of disease, exercise and sun exposure<0.01
Fitzgerald KC et al(25)	393 (39.5%) womenand 601 (60.4%) men	Q1 consumption AG: 61(7), 55 (10), 69 (3), 61 (9), 61 (5) Q2 consumption AG: 61(7), 54 (10), 69 (6), 60 (9), 62 (5) Q3 consumption AG: 61(7), 54 (10), 70 (6), 60 (9), 62 (5) Q4 consumption GA: 60 (7), 54 (10), 70 (6), 60 (9), 62 (5) Q5 consumption AG: 60.72 (7), 55 (10), 70.26 (6), 59 (9), 62(5)	No reference to
Huisman MHB et al (26)	Cases: 256 (38%) women and 428 (62%) men. Controls: 874 (41.8%) females and 1219 (58.2%) males	Cases: 62.4 (11.0) Controls: 62.6 (10.0)	P age: 0.69 P sex: 0.08 P exercise >0.05 P BMI, pre-diagnosis energy intake <0.05

Fondell E et al (27)	Q1 caffeine consumption: 155 (57.8%) females and 113 (42.2%) males Q2 caffeine consumption: 126 (51.09%) women and 116 (48.1%) men Q3 caffeine consumption: 148 (56.3%) females and 114 (43.7%) males Q4 caffeine consumption: 130 (49.9%) women and 131(50.1%) men Q5 caffeine consumption: 114 (46.3%) women and 132 (53.7%) men	Q1 caffeine consumption: 61.3 [8.7]. Q2 caffeine consumption: 60.8 [8.7]. Q3 caffeine consumption: 60.9 [8.5]. Q4 caffeine consumption: 60.8 [8.5]. Q5 caffeine consumption: 59.5 [8.3].	P sex-age trend: 0.58 P sex-age heterogeneity: 0.63
JinY et al (28)	Cases: 30 (41.7%) females and 42 (58.3%) males. Controls: 33 (45.8%) females and 39 (54.2%) men	Cases: 53.88 ± 10.02 years Controls: 53.35 ±14.49	P sex, age, height, tobacco, drink >0.05 P exercise, weight, BMI >0.05
Fondell Et al (29)	Q1 magnesium consumption : 120 (61%) women and76 (39%) men Q2 magnesium consumption: 116 (53.4%) females and 101 (46.6%) males Q3 magnesium consumption: 96 (48%) women and 104 (52%) men Q4 magnesium consumption:107 (43%) women and 142 (57%) men Q5 magnesium consumption: 85 (37%) women and 146 (63%) men	Q1 magnesium consumption: 59.9 (8.1) Q2 magnesium consumption: 59.9 (8.1) Q3 magnesium consumption: 59.9 (8.1) Q4 magnesium consumption: 59.9 (8.1) Q5 magnesium consumption: 59.9 (8.1)	P trend sex age: 0.46 P sex-age heterogeneity: 0.45

| **Fitzgerald KC et Al** (30) | 336 (30.75%) women and 757 (69.25%) men | Q1 carotenoids consumption: 45.9, 55.2, 59.9, 63.1, 61.7 years
Q2 carotenoid consumption: 46.4, 54.4, 59.1, 63.1, 61.7 years
Q3 carotenoid consumption: 47, 54.5, 59.9, 63.1, 61.6 years
Q4 carotenoids consumption: 47.1, 54.7, 60.8, 63.3, 61.6 years
Q5 carotenoid consumption: 47.7, 55.1, 61.4, 63.1, 61.6 years
Expressed as median | P sex-age trend: 0.003
P heterogeneity: 0.57 |

Table 4. Characteristics of the population

Regarding the characteristics of the study population, most of the studies had a higher percentage of men diagnosed with ALS, except in the papers by Fondell et al, Petimar et al and Lopes et al. As some papers expressed as patients in each age range and the rest as median, it was not possible to estimate the mean age of patients diagnosed with ALS from all studies together. In terms of the groups in each study, there were no significant differences, with the exception of the papers by Parkin et al, Lopes et al, Huisman et al and Fitzgerald et al, where there were significant differences in gender or age between the groups . There was no significant heterogeneity between the population in the pooled analyses of cohort studies.

Characteristics of the work interventions

All studies looked at intake or exposure to a micronutrient or dietary component, or even a type of diet, and its possible relationship to the risk of developing ALS or its prognosis if already diagnosed.

In all three RCTs patients received supplements or placebo depending on the group. In the most recent work by Dorst et al, patients were randomised into 4 groups and given calorie supplements; Group 1: Supplement with 405 kcal and 45 g fat per day (3*30 mL), Group 2: Supplement with 810 kcal and 90 g fat per day (30*3 mL), Group 3: Supplement with 900 kcal, 111.4 g carbohydrate, 35.3 g protein and 34.9 g fat (3*125 mL). Group 4: No supplement. The same supplementation as group 1 was given to patients in the intervention group in the work of Ludolph et al and the first paper by Dorst et al. In all three studies, patients assigned to placebo received 30 mL of placebo solution three times daily (equivalent to an additional fat intake of 0.1 g and an additional caloric intake of 8 kcal per day). These supplements were to be added to the usual diet, monitored by standardised questionnaires.

The other papers used frequency surveys and 24-hour dietary recall to estimate consumption.

For the estimation of mercury and W-3 PUFA consumption they used the species-specific mean mercury concentration or W-3 PUFA and multiplied this value by the frequency of consumption and servings.

For the assessment of fibre intake they divided the 5 most fibre-rich food groups: vegetables, fruits, grains, legumes and nuts/seeds and classified patients into tertiles of consumption.

Coffee consumption was determined using a validated food consumption frequency questionnaire. Two main groups of beverages were used for the analysis: total coffee (sum of grams per day of regular, decaffeinated and/or unidentified type) and total tea (sum of grams per day of caffeinated, caffeine-free and/or unidentified type of herbal tea). Results were expressed in tertiles of intake. This consumption was also analysed in a multicentre cross-sectional study in which patients with defined criteria were divided into non-consumers, current consumers and former consumers (subgroups according to number of cups).

To estimate alcohol exposure they divided patients with defined criteria into non-drinkers, former drinkers and current drinkers, who reported the number of alcoholic drinks per day and by type of drink (wine, beer and spirits). Drinking intensity (drinks/day) was estimated as the weighted average number of standard alcoholic units per day.

Several studies looked at exposure to numerous foods and nutrients simultaneously, or in a single form as in the case of zinc, magnesium, vitamin C and antioxidants. Mainly using a 24-hour recall collected by a dietitian nutritionist from patients or their caregivers. The questionnaires used differed between papers, both in number of questions and question design, generally using modified questionnaires between 63-200 items and adapted to each paper. Supplement consumption was not included in all studies when estimating antioxidant or micronutrient intake. The same method was used in the work of Huisman and Jin to detect differences between pre- and post-diagnosis intake patterns.

Main results

The main characteristics of the studies are included in Annex I: objectives, variables, results, limitations and conclusions of the studies.

The results of the studies were variable from study to study, although significant results were found for some nutrients and foods.

In the case of patients already diagnosed with ALS, foods were found that could affect survival and speed of progression of ALS; those options that increased survival included calorie supplements in some patient subgroups, intake of protein, fat, meat and dietary fibre, as well as intake of vitamins and antioxidants. Food items included vegetables, oils and condiments.

Factors decreasing survival or favouring progression included a deficit of intake, carbohydrate consumption, low zinc intake, long-term smoking or alcohol consumption.

On the other hand, the effect of tea or coffee was controversial, with a possible effect on disease progression.

On the other hand, foods and nutrients that could increase or decrease the risk of developing ALS and others whose consumption did not affect the risk of developing the disease were also observed.

The food group that increased the risk included red meat and processed pork and fast food. Also the consumption of total and animal protein, sodium, zinc, animal calcium, glutamic acid, total fat, saturated fat, trans fat and pre-disease cholesterol.

Among the nutrients with a protective effect, PUFA were detected, with W-3 PUFA being the most important, while there was no association with W-6. Some foods that significantly reduced the risk of developing the disease were wholemeal bread, vegetables or citrus fruits, vegetable calcium and beta-carotene or lutein. One study found a decreased risk with alcohol consumption.

Foods that did not affect the development of the disease included mercury, antioxidants, and magnesium intake.

The results for coffee and tea consumption on the risk of developing the disease were contradictory between studies, as was the case for fish.

DISCUSSION

The aim of this work was to elucidate the relationship between dietary habits and the risk of developing ALS or the evolution of ALS once established.

This review included papers that evaluated the effect of certain nutrients or foods on both the risk of developing the disease and the risk of developing the disease (12,13,18,20,25-30). (12,13,18,20,25-30) and on the evolution of the disease once it is established (11,14,15,17,19,21). (11,14,15,17,19,21-24). Common results regarding the effect of different foods and nutrients have been observed among most of the reviewed articles. Thus, the evidence demonstrates the importance, both before the development of the disease and at a more or less early stage of the disease course, of an adequate diet (31-33). The effect of food and nutrients achieved, in most of the articles reviewed, effects on the probability of developing ALS, as well as on the prognosis and survival from ALS (11,12,14-17,16). (11,12,14–17,20–26,28,30).

Some studies have analysed the role of dietary habits in disease, with contradictory results on the protective, detrimental or null role of some nutrients or foods (34-36). (34-36)The role of antioxidant and anti-inflammatory compounds, such as curcumin, carotenoids, vitamins, mainly from the B group, the ketogenic diet in reducing the progression of the disease, the harmful role of compounds such as glutamate, a diet rich in fats (not PUFA) or beta-methylalanine and the possible role of a diet rich in cholesterol, PUFA, purines and urate (34-36).

Mercury exposure, both environmental and through fish intake, has traditionally been considered a risk factor for the development of neurodegenerative diseases, including ALS, mainly by measuring the amount of mercury in nails as a biomarker in patients with and without ALS, obtaining higher levels in those patients with the disease (37,38). (37,38)however, the articles included in our review (12,13) found no relationship between its intake and the development of the disease.

With regard to PUFA consumption, the beneficial results on ALS risk found in our work (12,25) are in agreement with previous studies (39). (39) which also show a delay in the onset of the disease. A recent study, which investigated the possible causal relationship between some essential nutrients and the risk of ALS using Mendelian randomisation (MR) analysis, concluded that PUFA and fat-soluble vitamins are nutrients strongly related to the disease, demonstrating the importance of lipid metabolism in ALS (33). (33).

This review has included several papers that looked at coffee consumption on both the risk of developing the disease and the progression of the disease. (18,19,27)but no clear relationship was found in any of them, except in the work of Pupillo et al, in which a reduction in risk was observed (20). (20). These controversial results have been shown in other reviews before, in the review by Herden et Weissert, which included both animal and human research, with some of the studies included in our review finding a controversial effect of coffee, both protective and neutral as well as detrimental to ALS (40).

Articles using 24h recall questionnaires assessed the effect of various nutrients and foods and the two cross-sectional studies by Nieves et al. and Park et al. found a protective effect of wholemeal bread, raw vegetables and fruits and antioxidant micronutrients. Against intake of red meat, pork, protein, sodium, zinc and glutamic acid, total and saturated fats and cholesterol that were considered risk factors (20,23,24,26,28,30). Similar results in terms of protective effect of antioxidants and detrimental effect of saturated fatty acids and glutamic acid were observed as in other published reviews (31-33). Also common are the findings on magnesium intake and its lack of association with disease and the reviews cited above (29,34-36). (29,34-36).

In terms of higher calorie intake, the results of the included RCTs are similar to other published reviews on the subject (11,15,16). This is the case of the review by Pape et Grose, in which they concluded that diets that increase weight (such as high-fat or high-sugar and high-calorie diets) slow disease progression in both humans and mice, presumably by combating malnutrition due to hypermetabolism and disease progression (31). However, the ideal composition of this hypercaloric diet still needs to be elucidated. (31).

Yu et al, determined the effect of fibre intake on disease progression and cytokine levels. (14)while Pupillo et al. evaluated its effect on the risk of developing the disease (20). (20). In both cases, beneficial results were obtained in the subjects, which was confirmed in a mini-review article by Kuraszkiewicz et al , in which fibre intake was considered as an anti-ageing strategy that could decrease the risk of ALS and improve its progression. (32).

Kim et al. assessed macronutrient intake in early disease, finding that higher intakes of fat, protein and meat favoured longer-term survival (17). (17)(17), in contrast to the work of Pupillo et al, in which they were considered a risk factor for developing the disease (20). In this case, several studies have shown an association between increased meat protein intake and age-related diseases in the elderly population. In this case, Kuraszkiewicz et al. recommended following the World Health Organisation's recommendations for a healthy diet, postulating a restriction of free sugars and trans fats, including naturally occurring trans fats found in meat and dairy products from ruminant animals (32). The latter case also corroborates the results of the work of Nieves et al, in which they considered dairy products as a "bad food" and observed that it was associated with a worse ALSFR score (23). (23).

Similarly, in the work of Pupillo et al, it was concluded that zinc intake was a risk factor for the development of the disease (20), while Lopes et al, found a deficit of zinc intake in patients who had been diagnosed with ALS, in addition to a lower intake of energy and macronutrients (21). (21). Several studies have shown that some heavy metals such as cadmium and lead may be associated with an increased risk of developing ALS, however, they have also found that zinc has been found to have a lower risk depending on pre-disease blood metal levels, with lead appearing to increase risk the most (35).

In addition to nutrients, other lifestyle factors such as alcohol and tobacco use have been analysed in this review, and tobacco has previously been shown in case-control and longitudinal studies to increase the risk of developing ALS, as well as shortening survival in patients with ALS (41,42). (41,42). The latter effect was also observed in the work of Cucovici et al. (22). The case of alcohol has been more controversial, in the work of Huisman et al, the protective factor of alcohol was observed (26). (26)However, in the work of Cucovici et al. this effect was not clear, and was also associated with duration of consumption but not quantity (22). Other published studies concurred with the conclusions of Huisman et al, stating that alcohol could have a neuroprotective effect and reduce the risk of ALS (26,41,43). (26,41,43).

Highlight the controversial effect of some nutrients on both risk and established disease, for example, according to some manuscripts, vegetable consumption decreased the risk of developing ALS. (20)while in other papers (28) no such effect was found. Something similar occurred with proteins, which, although their consumption was associated with a longer survival time once the disease had developed, their consumption before the disease favoured the risk of developing the disease (17,20).

Published studies on dietary intervention in ALS patients conclude that early nutritional intervention is necessary, although it is recognised that patients are not adequately provided with it and often have nutritional deficits when treated in the clinic (44,45). (44,45)This may be due in part to the lack of consensus in the management of these patients, and the poorly established role of the dietitian nutritionist in their therapy (46). (46). De Marchi et al, proposed the use of technology to perform closer nutritional monitoring on these patients, in which patients recorded meals and received nutritional recommendations, with promising results in weight maintenance and BMI (47). Therefore, correct premorbid dietary habits and early nutritional intervention after diagnosis of the disease may be promising in the evolution of these patients.

LIMITATIONS

In interpreting the results of this review, it should be noted that most of the included studies were conducted with small sample sizes and were methodologically weak, with a minority of randomised clinical trials and several descriptive cross-sectional studies. In addition, there was no standardised approach to assessing the impact of diet on disease, as each study assessed different nutrients and foods, with a different methodology. Many variables could influence the results obtained from the different states, such as patient age, environmental conditions or genetic susceptibility, but also many other aspects linked to lifestyle and the interaction between the different variables, which cannot be understood with the design of the included studies. Another limitation encountered is the non-measurement of ALS incidence in the pooled analyses of cohort studies, however, patients were followed for long periods of time, and given their long follow-up, and the factor that patients diagnosed with ALS usually had a survival of 3-5 years after diagnosis, it was considered that no patients were lost, therefore, this limitation was corrected. All studies excluded patients with advanced disease (tracheostomy, ventilation), so the results obtained would only apply before developing the disease or in early stages.

CONCLUSIONS

The composition of the diet and intake of certain micronutrients and foods seems to influence the initial development and progression of ALS. Increased calorie intake may improve disease progression in certain subgroups of patients. Nutrients with antioxidant properties seem to decrease the risk of developing ALS and slow its progression. There is controversy in the results for some foods such as coffee or alcohol.

Knowledge of a dietary pattern and nutrients that prevent or delay the onset of ALS could be a method of primary prevention of ALS development in patients with risk factors. In addition, once the disease is established, in its early stages, an appropriate dietary pattern as a first line of treatment could be considered as a secondary prevention strategy, which would delay the progression of the disease, delaying more aggressive therapies such as tube feeding or parenteral nutrition.

However, the included studies analyse dietary components on an individual basis, which does not allow their adaptation to routine clinical practice. Studies in animal models and controlled clinical trials in humans with a larger number of patients and well-defined methodological criteria, dietary models and dietary guidelines are needed to allow us to compare results between them and establish the best model and recommendation for each type of patient. In this way, the true role of a specific dietary pattern in the prevention and treatment of ALS will be known.

On the other hand, greater access to a dietician-nutritionist from the earliest stages of the disease would be necessary in order to implement these guidelines.

BIBLIOGRAPHY

1. Masrori P, Van Damme P. Amyotrophic lateral sclerosis: a clinical review. Eur J Neurol. Oct 1, 2020;27(10):1918-29.

2. Longinetti E, Fang F. Epidemiology of amyotrophic lateral sclerosis: an update of recent literature. Curr Opin Neurol [Internet]. 2019;32(5). Available at: https://journals.lww.com/co-neurology/Fulltext/2019/10000/Epidemiology_of_amyotrophic_lateral_sclerosis__an.18.aspx

3. Štětkářová I, Ehler E. Diagnostics of Amyotrophic Lateral Sclerosis: Up to Date. Diagnostics. 2021;11(2).

4. Campanari ML, Bourefis AR, Kabashi E. Diagnostic Challenge and Neuromuscular Junction Contribution to ALS Pathogenesis. Front Neurol [Internet]. 2019;10. Available from: https://www.frontiersin.org/article/10.3389/fneur.2019.00068

5. Shen D, Yang X, Wang Y, He D, Sun X, Cai Z, et al. The Gold Coast criteria increases the diagnostic sensitivity for amyotrophic lateral sclerosis in a Chinese population. Transl Neurodegener. Dec 2021;10(1):28.

6. Cedarbaum JM, Stambler N, Malta E, Fuller C, Hilt D, Thurmond B, et al. The ALSFRS-R: a revised ALS functional rating scale that incorporates assessments of respiratory function. J Neurol Sci. October 1999;169(1-2):13-21.

7. Del Olmo García Mª D, Virgili Casas N, Cantón Blanco A, Lozano Fuster FM, Wanden-Berghe C, Avilés V, et al. Nutritional management of amyotrophic lateral sclerosis: summary of recommendations. Nutr Hosp. Oct 8, 2018;35(5):1243.

8. López-Gómez JJ, De Luis-Román DA. Nutritional support in the patient with amyotrophic lateral sclerosis: a systematic review. Nutr Clin EN Med. 4 May 2019;(1):53-71.

9. Quarracino C, Rey RC, Rodríguez GE. Amyotrophic lateral sclerosis (ALS): follow-up and treatment. Neurol Argent. April 2014;6(2):91-5.

10. Yoshino H. Edaravone for the treatment of amyotrophic lateral sclerosis. Expert Rev Neurother. Mar 4, 2019;19(3):185-93.

11. Dorst J, Doenz J, Kandler K, Dreyhaupt J, Tumani H, Witzel S, et al. Fat-rich versus carbohydrate-rich nutrition in ALS: a randomised controlled study. J Neurol Neurosurg Psychiatry. March 2022;93(3):298-302.

12. Hoffman HI, Bradley WG, Chen CY, Pioro EP, Stommel EW, Andrew AS. Amyotrophic Lateral Sclerosis Risk, Family Income, and Fish Consumption Estimates of Mercury and Omega-3 PUFAs in the United States. Int J Environ Res Public Health. 2021;18(9).

13. Parkin Kullmann J, Pamphlett R. A Comparison of Mercury Exposure from Seafood Consumption and Dental Amalgam Fillings in People with and without Amyotrophic Lateral Sclerosis (ALS): An International Online Case-Control Study. Int J Environ Res Public Health. Dec 14, 2018;15(12):2874.

14. Yu H, Kim SH, Noh MY, Lee S, Park Y. Relationship between Dietary Fiber Intake and the Prognosis of Amytrophic Lateral Sclerosis in Korea. Nutrients. Nov 7, 2020;12(11):3420.

15. Dorst J, Schuster J, Dreyhaupt J, Witzel S, Weishaupt JH, Kassubek J, et al. Effect of high-caloric nutrition on serum neurofilament light chain levels in amyotrophic lateral sclerosis. J Neurol Neurosurg Psychiatry. September 2020;91(9):1007-9.

16. Ludolph AC, Dorst J, Dreyhaupt J, Weishaupt JH, Kassubek J, Weiland U, et al. Effect of High-Caloric Nutrition on Survival in Amyotrophic Lateral Sclerosis. Ann Neurol. Feb 1, 2020;87(2):206-16.

17. Kim B, Jin Y, Kim SH, Park Y. Association between macronutrient intake and amyotrophic lateral sclerosis prognosis. Nutr Neurosci. Jan 2, 2020;23(1):8-15.

18. Petimar J, O'Reilly É, Adami H -O., Brandt PA, Buring J, English DR, et al. Coffee, tea, and caffeine intake and amyotrophic lateral sclerosis mortality in a pooled analysis of eight prospective cohort studies. Eur J Neurol. March 2019;26(3):468-75.

19. Cucovici A, Ivashynka A, Fontana A, Russo S, Mazzini L, Mandrioli J, et al. Coffee and Tea Consumption Impact on Amyotrophic Lateral Sclerosis Progression: A Multicenter Cross-Sectional Study. Front Neurol. July 28, 2021;12:637939.

20. Pupillo E, Bianchi E, Chiò A, Casale F, Zecca C, Tortelli R, et al. Amyotrophic lateral sclerosis and food intake. Amyotroph Lateral Scler Front Degener. Apr 3, 2018;19(3-4):267-74.

21. Lopes da Silva HF, Araújo Brito AN, Silva de Freitas EP, Teixeira Dourado Jr ME, Sena-Evangelista KCM, Leite Lais L. Dietary intake and zinc status in amyotrophic lateral sclerosis. Nutr Hosp [Internet]. October 27, 2017 [cited Mar 16, 2022]; Available from: http://revista.nutricionhospitalaria.net/index.php/nh/article/view/1004.

22. Cucovici A, Fontana A, Ivashynka A, Russo S, Renna V, Mazzini L, et al. The Impact of Lifetime Alcohol and Cigarette Smoking Loads on Amyotrophic Lateral Sclerosis Progression: A Cross-Sectional Study. Life. Apr 17, 2021;11(4):352.

23. Nieves JW, Gennings C, Factor-Litvak P, Hupf J, Singleton J, Sharf V, et al. Association Between Dietary Intake and Function in Amyotrophic Lateral Sclerosis. JAMA Neurol. Dec 1, 2016;73(12):1425.

24. Park Y, Park J, Kim Y, Baek H, Kim SH. Association between nutritional status and disease severity using the amyotrophic lateral sclerosis (ALS) functional rating scale in ALS patients. Nutrition. Nov 1, 2015;31(11):1362-7.

25. Fitzgerald KC, O'Reilly ÉJ, Falcone GJ, McCullough ML, Park Y, Kolonel LN, et al. Dietary ω-3 Polyunsaturated Fatty Acid Intake and Risk for Amyotrophic Lateral Sclerosis. JAMA Neurol. Sep 1, 2014;71(9):1102.

26. Huisman MHB, Seelen M, Doormaal PTC van, Jong SW de, Vries JHM de, Kooi AJ van der, et al. Effect of Presymptomatic Body Mass Index and Consumption of Fat and Alcohol on Amyotrophic Lateral Sclerosis. JAMA Neurol. 2015;72 10:1155-62.

27. Fondell E, O'Reilly ÉiJ, Fitzgerald KC, Falcone GJ, Kolonel LN, Park Y, et al. Intakes of caffeine, coffee and tea and risk of amyotrophic lateral sclerosis: Results from five cohort studies. Amyotroph Lateral Scler Front Degener. Aug 27, 2015;16(5-6):366-71.

28. Jin Y, Oh K, Oh S il, Baek H, Kim SH, Park Y. Dietary intake of fruits and beta-carotene is negatively associated with amyotrophic lateral sclerosis risk in Koreans: A case-control study. Nutr Neurosci. Apr 1, 2014;17(3):104-8.

29. Fondell E, O'Reilly ÉJ, Fitzgerald KC, Falcone GJ, McCullough ML, Park Y, et al. Magnesium intake and risk of amyotrophic lateral sclerosis: Results from five large cohort studies. Amyotroph Lateral Scler Front Degener. September 2013;14(5-6):356-61.

30. Fitzgerald KC, O'Reilly ÉJ, Fondell E, Falcone GJ, McCullough ML, Park Y, et al. Intakes of vitamin C and carotenoids and risk of amyotrophic lateral sclerosis: Pooled results from 5 cohort studies: Carotenoids and ALS. Ann Neurol. February 2013;73(2):236-45.

31. Pape JA, Grose JH. The effects of diet and sex in amyotrophic lateral sclerosis. Rev Neurol (Paris). May 1, 2020;176(5):301-15.

32. Kuraszkiewicz B, Goszczyńska H, Podsiadły-Marczykowska T, Piotrkiewicz M, Andersen P, Gromicho M, et al. Potential Preventive Strategies for Amyotrophic Lateral Sclerosis. Front Neurosci [Internet]. 2020;14. Available from: https://www.frontiersin.org/article/10.3389/fnins.2020.00428

33. Xia K, Wang Y, Zhang L, Tang L, Zhang G, Huang T, et al. Dietary-Derived Essential Nutrients and Amyotrophic Lateral Sclerosis: A Two-Sample Mendelian Randomization Study. Nutrients.

2022;14(5).

34. D'Amico E, Grosso G, Nieves JW, Zanghì A, Factor-Litvak P, Mitsumoto H. Metabolic Abnormalities, Dietary Risk Factors and Nutritional Management in Amyotrophic Lateral Sclerosis. Nutrients. 2021;13(7).

35. D'Antona S, Caramenti M, Porro D, Castiglioni I, Cava C. Amyotrophic Lateral Sclerosis: A Diet Review. Foods. 2021;10(12).

36. Goncharova PS, Davydova TK, Popova TE, Novitsky MA, Petrova MM, Gavrilyuk OA, et al. Nutrient Effects on Motor Neurons and the Risk of Amyotrophic Lateral Sclerosis. Nutrients. 2021;13(11).

37. Andrew AS, O'Brien KM, Jackson BP, Sandler DP, Kaye WE, Wagner L, et al. Keratinous biomarker of mercury exposure associated with amyotrophic lateral sclerosis risk in a nationwide U.S. study. Amyotroph Lateral Scler Front Degener. August 2020;21(5-6):420-7.

38. Andrew AS, Chen CY, Caller TA, Tandan R, Henegan PL, Jackson BP, et al. Toenail mercury Levels are associated with amyotrophic lateral sclerosis risk. Muscle Nerve. July 1, 2018;58(1):36-41.

39. Veldink JH, Kalmijn S, Groeneveld GJ, Wunderink W, Koster A, de Vries JHM, et al. Intake of polyunsaturated fatty acids and vitamin E reduces the risk of developing amyotrophic lateral sclerosis. J Neurol Neurosurg Amp Psychiatry. April 1, 2007;78(4):367.

40. Herden L, Weissert R. The Impact of Coffee and Caffeine on Multiple Sclerosis Compared to Other Neurodegenerative Diseases. Front Nutr [Internet]. 2018;5. Available from: https://www.frontiersin.org/article/10.3389/fnut.2018.00133

41. de Jong SW, Huisman MHB, Sutedja NA, van der Kooi AJ, de Visser M, Schelhaas HJ, et al. Smoking, Alcohol Consumption, and the Risk of Amyotrophic Lateral Sclerosis: A Population-based Study. Am J Epidemiol. Aug 1, 2012;176(3):233-9.

42. Wang H, O'Reilly ÉJ, Weisskopf MG, Logroscino G, McCullough ML, Thun MJ, et al. Smoking and Risk of Amyotrophic Lateral Sclerosis: A Pooled Analysis of 5 Prospective Cohorts. Arch Neurol. 2011 Feb 1;68(2):207-13.

43. E M, Yu S, Dou J, Jin W, Cai X, Mao Y, et al. Association between alcohol consumption and amyotrophic lateral sclerosis: a meta-analysis of five observational studies. Neurol Sci. Aug 1, 2016;37(8):1203-8.

44. Carrera Juliá S, Catarina-Moreira A, Adriana-Santos C, Fonseca J, Drehmer E. Nutritional intake in patients affected by amyotrophic lateral sclerosis in an outpatient artificial nutrition clinic in Portugal.

Rev Esp Nutr Human Dietetics. Dec 28, 2021;25(4):353-64.

45. White S, Zarotti N, Beever D, Bradburn M, Norman P, Coates E, et al. The nutritional management of people living with amyotrophic lateral sclerosis: A national survey of dietitians. J Hum Nutr Diet. Dec 1, 2021;34(6):1064-71.

46. Essat M, Coates E, Clowes M, Beever D, Hackney G, White S, et al. Understanding the current nutritional management for people with amyotrophic lateral sclerosis - A mapping review. Clin Nutr ESPEN [Internet]. March 21, 2022; Available from: https://www.sciencedirect.com/science/article/pii/S240545772200208X.

47. De Marchi F, Amantea IA, Serioli M, Sulis E, Boella G, Alloatti F, et al. E-health solutions for amyotrophic lateral sclerosis patients: A chatbot for dietary monitoring. J Neurol Sci [Internet]. October 1, 2021 [cited April 17, 2022];429. Available from: https://doi.org/10.1016/j.jns.2021.119386

ANNEX I: OBJECTIVES, VARIABLES, RESULTS, LIMITATIONS AND CONCLUSIONS

Author	Target	Variables	Results	P	Limitations	Conclusion
Dorst e t al (11)	Determine in hypercaloric supplements which nutrient composition offers optimal tolerability and weight gain. optimal tolerability and weight gain.	Primary endpoint: tolerability (incidence of adverse effects) Secondary endpoints: change in from weight change, consumption habits, change in ALS scales.	Gastrointestinal Gastrointestinal side effects were more frequent in the UHCFS group (75.0%), while loss of appetite was more frequent in the UHCCS group (35.3%). Patients gained +0.9 kg/month of body weight (IQR -0.9 to 1.5) in the HCFS group. +0.9 kg/month (IQR -0.8 to 2.0) in the UHCFS group. +0.6 kg/month (IQR -0.3 to 1.9) in the UHCCS group. -0.5 kg/month, (IQR -1.4 to 1.3) in the unsupplemented group.	p=0.03 p=0.05 p=0.08 p=0.42	Little study time. Weight changes were assessed with respect to the anamnesis (inaccurate). Slight differences between the study population.	Calorie supplements may cause mild to moderate tolerability problems in ALS patients, particularly gastrointestinal problems with high-fat supplements and loss of appetite with carbohydrate-rich supplements. The supplements studied were suitable to increase the weight body.

Hoffman HI et al (12)	Determine whether mercury exposure through fish consumption patterns increases the **risk** of ALS.	Annual consumption of mercury. Annual consumption of omega-3 PUFA.	Household income showed a positive association with ALS risk. Neither the estimated annual intake of mercury and omega-3 polyunsaturated fatty acids through fish and seafood consumption were associated with the risk of ALS.	(p = 0,0003, adjusted) P= 0.82 and P= 0.74	Self-reported dietary recall with frequencies (weekly, monthly) and type of fish (inaccurate) Retrospective data recording. Variable mercury concentrations in fish. Results do not generalisable to other stocks Biases in the answers.	Fish and seafood consumption was not a risk factor for ALS. Protective effect of PUFAs. The incidence of ALS was related to socio-economic status.

Parkin JA et al (13)	Determine whether exposure to mercury through fish and dental amalgam consumption patterns increases the risk of ALS.	Frequency of seafood consumption. Food favourite seafood. μg of mercury exposure per month from seafood. Mercury contained in fillings.	No differences were observed between cases and controls in the distribution of mercury exposure in their favourite seafood. The mean monthly mercury exposure value was slightly lower in ALS respondents (39 μg per month versus 49 μg per month for controls) but these values did not differ significantly.	P= 0.13	Problems associated with the use of surveys online. Female respondents with ALS were older than their female controls. The mercury content of all shellfish could not be determined.	Exposure to mercury from seafood or mercury-containing dental fillings was no more common in people with ALS than in controls.

| **Yu et al** (14) | To investigate whether the intake of different types of dietary fibre is related to the **rate** of disease **progression (ΔFS) and survival time.** progression rate (ΔFS) and survival time.

To examine whether dietary fibre intake was correlated with cytokine levels in cerebrospinal fluid (CSF) of ALS patients. | Fibre intake

Cytokine levels

Occurrence of event: PEG, Tracheostomy or death

Disease progression

Survival | Lower than average disease progression was observed in higher tertiles of plant fibre intake.

Participants in the highest tertile for plant fibre consumption showed more survival in the Kaplan-Meier analysis.

Vegetable fibre intake correlates negatively with pro-inflammatory cytokines (interleukin IL-1β, interleukin with proinflammatory cytokines (interleukin IL-1β, IL-6 and monocyte chemoattractant protein-1 levels) in cerebrospinal fluid, IL-6 and monocyte chemoattractant protein-1 levels) in cerebrospinal fluid. | P<0.001

P= 0.033 | Fibre intake was measured only at the time of the survey, it may not reflect long-term intake.

Only 27 CSF samples were available for cytokine analysis; the findings may not be representative.

Adjustments were made for confounding factors, unmeasured factors could have affected the results. | The intake of plant fibre intake could influence the rate of disease progression and survival time in Korean ALS patients.

In addition, plant fibre intake was negatively correlated with pro-inflammatory cytokines, suggesting that plant fibre intake may delay disease progression. pro-inflammatory cytokines, suggesting that plant fibre intake may delay disease progression and prolong survival time. and prolong survival time in Korean ALS patients through an effect |

anti-inflammatory.

Dorst et al (15)	To investigate the effect of a high-fat diet on serum Nfl levels, using blood samples.	Level of neurofilaments in the blood.	Serum NfL levels were positively associated with the rate of progression at baseline (rho=0.57) as well as during the intervention (rho=0.71).	P<0.01	Low number of samples available	The results of the NfL analysis in ALS patients treated with HCFD or placebo indicated that serum NfL values can serve as as prognostic biomarker to improve patient stratification and as a complementary outcome parameter in addition to survival and ALSFRS- R.
		Difference between the levels of neurofilaments in the blood between several various points.	Those who progressed rapidly had higher median baseline NfL (132.5 pg/mL, IQR 79.0- 243.0) compared to those who progressed slowly (72.0 pg/mL, IQR 47.0-104.0).	P<0.01	Few patients per subgroup	
		Disease progression of the disease				
		Survival	Patients on placebo showed an increase in NfL with a median positive slope of 0.51 (-0.44 -2.17) pg/mL per month, while patients in the high calorie fat diet (HCFD) group showed a decrease in serum NfL levels with a median negative slope of -0.61 (-2.87 to -1.15) pg/mL per month.	P=0.02		
				P= 0.043		

This effect was mainly caused by patients who progressed fast, with HCFD (-1.22pg/ml (-3.14-0.85); n=17) and
placebo (+3.7pg/mL (0.0-9.29; n=10; P= 0.002 p=0.03) within this subgroup, but not in the slow ones.

The statistical model confirmed an effect of HCFD on serum NfL levels for the whole population.

In the subgroup of patients with high NfL (n=25), the overall survival of HCFD-treated patients (n=11) was prolonged compared to placebo (n=14).

P= 0.01

On placebo, the probability of survival at 18 months was 0.21 (95% CI 0.03 to 0.49),

0.67 (95% CI 0.28 to 0.88) in the HCFD group. The HR was 0.21, bilateral 95% CI 0.05 to 0.82.

| Ludolph AC et al (16) | To assess the effectiveness of an HCFD for to increase survival in ALS patients. | Primary endpoint: survival time

Variables secondary variables: change in ALSFRS-R, vital capacity, quality of life

vital capacity, quality of life

Time to tracheostomy or death

Change from weight

Occurrenceof adverse effects or alterations in clinical or laboratory | Survival analysis showed a survival probability of 0.39 (95%CI = 0.27-0.51) in the placebo group and 0.37 (95%CI = 0.25-049) in the HCFD group, both after 28 months (time point of last event).

The hazard ratio was 0.97, one-sided 97.5% CI = -∞ to 1.44. | P= 0.44 | Not knowing whether the result is due to more calories or more fat

Low compliance | The results did not provide evidence of a life-prolonging effect of the HCFD for all ALS patients. However, post hoc analysis revealed a significant survival benefit for the subgroup of patients with rapid progression. |

		parameters. laboratory parameters.				

| Kim B et al (17) | To investigate whether macronutrient intakes in early ALS were positively associated with survival and duration from from symptom onset to death, tracheostomy or non-invasive ventilation (NIV). | Time to death, tracheostomy or NIV. Nutrient intake and food | ALS patients were classified as short-term group (n=79) and long-term group (n=69) according to mean survival time (33.03±14.01 months). Short-term survival was negatively associated with fat, protein, and meat intake, and positively associated with carbohydrate intake after adjustment for confounders. Survival time was positively associated with fat, protein and meat intake, but not associated with carbohydrate intake. | P Fats: 0.039 P Protein: 0.032 P Meat: 0.003 P HC: 0.016 | Small sample size and exclusion of patients who did not reach the endpoint could cause selection bias. Intake was measured with 24-hour recall only once, which may not have been sufficient to determine usual intake. sufficient to determine usual intake. The dietary survey could not be conducted after symptom onset due to diagnostic delay and outpatient visit | The present study suggested that increased intake of fats and proteins, particularly meat in the early stages of the disease, could prolong survival in ALS patients. |

interval.

Possible confounding factors.

Petimar J et al (18)	To determi ne the associations between coffee, tea and caffeine intake and the **risk** of ALS mortality.	Coffee, tea and caffeine intake Time to death or loss of tracking	No statistically significant associations were observed between coffee, tea or caffeine intake and the risk of ALS mortality. The pooled multivariate RR (MVRR) for ≥3 cups per day vs. >0 to <1 cup per day was 1.04 (95%CI: 0.74-1.47) for coffee and 1.17 (95%CI: 0.77-1.79) for tea. The combined MVRR comparing the highest to the lowest tertile of caffeine intake (mg/day) was 0.99 (95% CI 0.80 -1.23). Nose no statistically significant results were observed statistically significant results were not observed when the exposures were modelled as	P>0.05	Low power of detection. Nose duration or history of caffeine exposure or changes over time could not be examined. Data collection differed between the studies. Only data on ALS deaths, not on new cases.	There are no associations between coffee, tea or total caffeine intake and risk of ALS mortality.

tertiles or

continuously.

| **Cucovici A et al** (19) | To know the influence of coffee and tea consumption on the rate of **progression of** ALS. | Coffee consumption

Progression of the disease | Current coffee consumers were 179 (74.3%), 34 (14.1%) were non-consumers, and 22 (9.1%) were ex-consumers, while 6 (2.5%) consumed decaffeinated.

Disease progression correlated weakly with the duration of coffee consumption, but not with the number of cup-years, nor with the intensity of coffee consumption (cups/day).

Current tea consumers numbered 101 (41.9%), 6 (2.5%) were ex-consumers, and 134 (55.6%) were non-consumers.

Among current and former consumers, 27 (25.2%) consumed only green tea, 51 (47.7%) consumed only black tea and 29 (27.1%) consumed both. | P= 0.034

P= 0.028 | Recall bias

Possible influence of other variables | Tea or coffee consumption was not associated with the rate of ALS progression. |

The progression of the disease is
correlated weakly with the duration of
black tea consumption.

Pupillo et al (20)	Check whether specific foods and nutrients could be **risk factors or protective factors** for ALS.	Daily intake of macronutrients, micronutrients and energy. and energy. Development of ALS	Risk reduction was found for coffee and tea (OR ¼ 0.29, 95 % CI 0.14- 0.60), wholemeal bread (OR ¼ 0.55, 95 % CI 0.31- 0.99), raw vegetables (OR ¼ 0.25, 95 % CI 0.13- 0.52) and citrus fruits (OR ¼ 0.49, 95 % CI 0.25 0.97). An increased risk was observed for red meat (OR ¼ 2.96, 95 % CI 1.46-5.99) and pork and processed meat (OR ¼ 3.87, 95 % CI 1.86-8.07). An increased risk was found for total protein (OR ¼ 2.96, 95 % CI 1.08-8.10), animal protein (OR ¼ 2.91, 95 % CI 1.33-6.38), sodium (OR ¼ 3.96, 95 % CI 1.45-10.84), zinc (OR ¼ 2.78, 95 % CI 1.01-7.83) and glutamic acid (OR ¼ 3.63, 95 % CI 1.08-12.2).	P coffee and tea: 0.0079 P pan: 0.0323 P vegetables: 0.0005 P fruit: 0.0198 P red meat: 0.006 P pork: 0.006 P prot tot: 0.0437 P prot animal: 0.007 P Na: 0.00587 P Zn: 0.027 P glutamic: 0.0684	Difference between the Italian diet and other diets. Inherent biases in case-control design. Reverse causality. Dietary changes during the course of the disease.	Some foods/nutrients may be risk factors and some may be protective factors for ALS.

Lopes HE al (21)	Assess intake dietary and zinc status in ALS patients.	IngestadeZinc , energy, proteins, fats and carbohydrates. Zincurinary and in plasma.	Average energy intake, protein, carbohydrates and fat was significantly lower for the case group. There was a higher prevalence of inadequate zinc intake in the case group (35%) compared to controls (27%). Mean plasma zinc was significantly lower in the case group than in the controls (77.13 ± 22.21 vs 87.84 ± 22.21). 17.44 µg Zn/dl). Urinary zinc did not differ significantly between cases and controls. In the case group, plasma and urine zinc concentrations were below reference values in 50.0% and 52.6% of patients,	Protein <0.001 HC: <0.001 Fats: <0.001 P= 0.897 P= 0.05 P= 0.155	Low number of patients	Compared to the control group, patients with ALS showed lower intakes of energy and macronutrients, higher prevalence of inadequate zinc intake, lower plasma zinc concentration, as well as a tendency to decrease urinary zinc excretion.

respectively

Cucovici A et al (22)	To determine the influence of tobacco and alcohol use on rates of ALS progression. ALS progression.	Disease progression rate Exposure to tobacco and of alcohol ALS progression.	Current smokers accounted for 44 (18.3%) participants, ex-smokers accounted for 10 (4.1%) and non-smokers accounted for 10 (4.1%). smokers accounted for 187 (77.6%). The age of ALS onset was lower in current smokers than in non-smokers, and the ΔFS was slightly, but not significantly, higher for smokers of >14 cigarettes/day. Drinkers accounted for 147 (61.0%) participants, ex-drinkers accounted for 5 (2.1%) and non-drinkers accounted for 89 (36.9%). Log(ΔFS) correlated weakly only with drinking duration, but not with mean drinks/day or drink-year.	P= 0.406 P= 0.028	Intrinsic limitations a cross-sectional design that prevents the establishment of a causal link. Occurrence of other potential confounding variables.	Possible secondary role of smoking in of smoking in worsening disease progression. A possible interaction with alcohol consumption was suggested.

| Nieves JW et al (23) | To assess associations between nutrients, individually and in groups, and function in ALS and respiratory function at diagnosis. | ALSFRS- R score

Nutrient intake

Capacity

Fo
rced Vital Capacity (FVC) | Higher intake of antioxidants and carotenoids was associated with higher ALSFRS-R scores or percentage FVC.

Using a statistical method, it was observed that 'good' micronutrients and 'good' food groups were positively associated with ALSFRS-R scores (β [SE], 2.7 [0.69] and 2.9 [0.9], respectively) and FVC percentages (β [SE], 12.1 [2.8] and 11.5 [3.4], respectively).

Positive associations were found in ALSFRS-R (β [SE], 1.5 [0.61]; P = .02) and in CVF (β [SE], 5.2 [2.2]; for selected vitamins in exploratory analyses. | P<0.001

P= 0.02 | Nose partnerships could not be established

Small sample size

Data collection survey

Possible misallocation of nutrients | The association between initial dietary intake and ALS severity (as assessed by percentage of FVC and by percentage of FVC and ALSFRS-R ALSFRS-R score) indicated a consistent association between these variables y certain nutrients.

Antioxidant nutrients, foods rich in rich carotenoid- and fibre-rich foods and vegetable consumption were associated with better ALS function |

using 2 different analysis methods.

| Park Y et al (24) | To investigate the hypothesis that nutritional status is negatively associated with disease severit y using the ALSFRS-R. | ALSFRS- R score

Dietary intake

BMI, Geriatric Nutritional Risk Index (GNRI) | BMI and GNRI were significantly lower in patients in the lowest ALSFRS-R tertile.

BMI and GNRI were also correlated with ALSFRS-R score, bulbar score, albumin levels, total score, lymphocyte count and total daily energy expenditure.

Intakes of energy and most nutrients were significantly lower than for were significantly lower in patients in the lowest tertiles of ALSFRS-R, but the significance disappeared after adjusting for energy intake.

Intakes of vegetables, grains, condiments, and oils were also significantly lower in patients in the lowest tertile of | $P < 0.001$

Vegetables: 0.013

Grains: 0.012

Seasonings : 0.02 | The cross-sectional design was unable to establish cause-effect relationships.

Possible confounding factors.

Only patients with mild to moderate stage were included. | Nutritional status, as assessed by BMI and GNRI, was negatively associated with disease severity using ALSFRS-R.

Nutrient intake decreased with disease progression in ALS patients.

i n ALS patients. |

			ALSFRS-R.	Oils: 0.07		

Fitzgerald KC et al (25)	Browse the association between consumptio n of ω6 and ω-3 PUFA and the risk of ALS.	Diagnosis of ALS Time to death Intake of each nutrient	A higher intake of ω-3 PUFA was associated with a reduced risk of ALS. The adjusted RR for the highest to lowest quintile was 0.66 (95% CI, 0.53-0.81). Consumption of α-linolenic acid (RR, 0.73; 95% CI, 0.59-0.89) and ω-3 PUFA (RR, 0.84; 95%CI, 0.65- 1.08) were inversely associated. Intake of ω-6 PUFA was not associated with risk of ALS.	P< 0.001 P= 0.003 P= 0.03	Use of death instead of incidence. Bias in favour of survivors. Identification of cases through death certificates death certificat es with possible misclassification errors Error at the estimation of the intake.	Eating foods o f foods rich in ω-3 PUFA may help prevent or delay the onset of ALS.

| Huisman MHB et al (26) | Determine the association between premorbid dietary intake y the **risk** of sporadic ALS. | Energy and nutrient intake

BMI

Survival

Risk

o

f disease | The mean pre-symptomatic total daily energy intake was higher in cases compared to controls (2258 [730] vs. to 2119 [619] kcal/day.

Presymptomatic body mass index was lower in cases (25.7 [4.0] vs. 26.0 [3.7]).

Higher premorbid intakes of total fat (OR 1.14, 1.07-1.23), saturated fat (OR 1.43, 1.25-1.64), trans-fatty acids (OR 1.03, 1.01- 1.05), and cholesterol (OR 1.08, 1.05- 1.12) were associated with an increased risk of ALS.

Higher alcohol intake (OR 0.91, 0.84-0.99) was associated with a decreased risk of ALS.

These associations were independent of total energy intake, age, sex, body mass index, educational level, smoking and physical activity. No | P<0.01

P= 0.02

P<0.001

P= 0.03 | Bias

r

ecall bias

Possible effect of disease diagnosis on dietary habits. | The combination of a positive association between low BMI and high premorbid fat intake suggested increased resting energy expenditure prior to clinical onset of ALS. |

significant associations were found between total energy intake, age, sex, body mass index, educational level, smoking and physical activity.

diet and survival.

Fondell E et al (27)	To examine the association between caffeine, coffee and tea consumption and ALS **risk.**	Diagnosis of AS Consumption of coffee, tea and caffeine (cups and grams).	Caffeine intake was not associated with risk of ALS; the multivariable adjusted pooled RR comparing highest to lowest intake quintile was 0.96 (95% CI 0.81-1.16). Similarly, neither coffee 1.00 (95%CI 0.82-1.22), nor tea 0.99 (95% CI 0.79-1.23) were associated with the risk of ALS.	P= 0.66 P= 0.98 P= 0.42	Use death instead of incidence. Possible errors in the estimation of consumption.	The results of this study did not support the association of caffeine or caffeinated beverages with risk of ALS.
Jin Y et al (28)	To investigate the hypothesis that fruit intake, rich in antioxidant nutrients, is negatively associated with ALS risk.	Dietary intake Development of ALS	Fruit consumption was negatively associated with ALS risk, but beef, fish and fast food intake were positively associated with ALS risk. Furthermore, the risk of ALS was negatively associated with intake of vegetable calcium and beta-carotene, while it was positively associated with intake of total calcium and animal calcium. Intake of vegetables and other	P<0 .001 for Ca animal, beef and fast food P fruit: 0.004 P fish: 0.002 P plant calcium: 0.005, β-carotene: 0.013	Small sample size. Cross-sectional design that did not allow cause-effect relationships to be established. No changes in dietary habits were detected.	Fruit and beta-carotene intake decreased the risk of developing ALS.

| | | | antioxidant nutrients had no effect. | Total P ca: 0.024 | Recall bias in the questionnaires. | |

Fondell E et al (29)	Explore the relationship between dietary intake of magnesium and the **risk** of ALS	Magnesium intake Calcium intake Diagnosis of ALS	There was no association between dietary magnesium intake and risk of ALS (multivariable adjusted RR 1.07, 95%CI: 0.88-1.31). comparing the highest to the lowest quintile in the pooled analyses. Results were similar between cohorts (data not shown) and between men and women (men: RR 1.10, 95%CI: 0.85-1.41; women: RR 1.08, IC95%: 0.71-1.64).	P= 0.3	Mortality rather than incidence was used as a proxy for ALS. No changes in dietary magnesium intake were taken into account. Possible misestimation of intake when using reminders. Lack of information on the use of supplements.	No protective effect of magnesium intake on the risk of developing ALS was observed.

Fitzgerald KC et al (30).	Investigate the relationship between vitamin C and carotenoid intake and **risk** of ALS.	Deathby ALS Diagnosis from ALS Vitamin C intake Intake of carotenoids	Higher carotenoid intake was associated with a lower risk of ALS (pooled RR, multivariable adjusted for highest to lowest quintile: 0.75; 95%CI: 0.61-0.91). The highest dietary intakes of β-carotene and lutein were inversely inversely with risk of ALS. The pooled multivariate RRs comparing the highest to the lowest quintile for β-carotene and lutein were 0.85 (95% CI 0.64-1.13 and 0.79 (95% CI 0.64-0.96) respectively. Lycopene, β-cryptoxanthin and vitamin C were associated with a reduced risk of ALS.	P trend = 0,004 P trend = 0.03 P trend= 0.01 P> 0.05	Use of death rather than incidence of ALS in some studies Influence of ALS on dietary habits. Possible changes in dietary habits.	Eating foods rich in carotenoids may help prevent or delay the onset of ALS.

Table 5. Results and conclusions

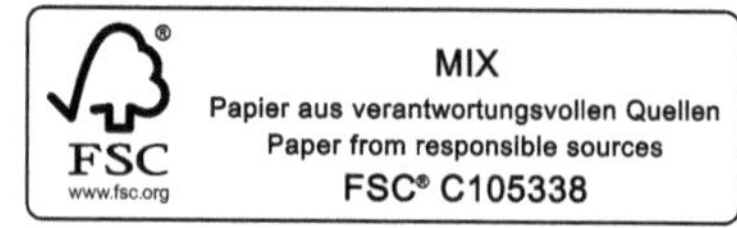

Printed by Books on Demand GmbH, Norderstedt / Germany